Overcoming Com

Dr Dawn's Guide to Women's Health

DR DAWN HARPER

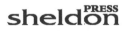

First published in Great Britain in 2015

Sheldon Press
36 Causton Street
London SW1P 4ST
www.sheldonpress.co.uk

British Library Cataloguing-in-Publication Data
A catalogue record for this book is available from the British Library

ISBN 978-1-84709-354-7
eBook ISBN 978-1-84709-355-4

Typeset by Fakenham Prepress Solutions, Fakenham, Norfolk NR21 8NN
First printed in Great Britain by Ashford Colour Press
Subsequently digitally reprinted in Great Britain

eBook by Fakenham Prepress Solutions, Fakenham, Norfolk NR21 8NN

Produced on paper from sustainable forests

To my agent, Debbie Catchpole,
without whom this series would never have got off the ground

Contents

Note to the reader

This is not a medical book and is not intended to replace advice from your doctor. Consult your pharmacist or doctor if you believe you have any of the symptoms described, and if you think you might need medical help.

Introduction

When I was 12 years old, I was admitted to hospital with appendicitis. In those days, after the operation you stayed in hospital for a few days and, as I recuperated, I found I was fascinated with what the doctors and nurses were doing. By the time I was discharged, my decision was made – I wanted to be a doctor. Three years later, when careers advice was being handed out, I steadfastly refused to discuss anything else. I knew what I wanted to do and, like any self-respecting 15 year old, I knew much better than the adults around me! Finally, my headmistress called a meeting with my parents. She was concerned I was making a mistake. She told them I was a linguist, not a scientist, and that if, jointly, they could persuade me to rethink, I would have a very bright career ahead of me. Thank goodness they failed! I am lucky to love my job, all aspects of it, although I do have to concede that my teachers may have had a point as my working week today involves more time talking and writing about medical issues than it does actually practising them. In fact, when I wrote my first book in 2007, I dedicated it to my German teacher who I still see every year.

So what happened, and how did I get to where I am today? Well, fast forward a few years and I qualified in medicine at Charing Cross and Westminster Medical School. I still remember the day that I called home and simply said 'It's Dr Harper speaking'. I felt on top of the world. To this day every time I drive into London (which is very often!), I look right at the Charing Cross hospital in Fulham with fond memories. After I qualified I spent a number of years working in various medical specialties and took post-graduate exams to become a member of the Royal College of Physicians. I then spent some time working in Australia. They have a wonderful medical system, but it is not *free for all* as it is here in the UK, and, for the first time, I started to appreciate the real cost of treatment and just how wonderful our NHS is. I often say that the NHS is 'like your Mum' – she may not be perfect, but she has your best interests at heart and, one thing is for sure, you will miss her when she is gone. I hope that day never comes, but I do believe we all have a responsibility to look after her.

I have a responsibility as an individual, as a mother and as a doctor and broadcaster, to make sure that my family, my patients, my viewers and my readers are in the best position possible to understand any medical problems they have, and know what they can do to help themselves, which is one of the reasons I wanted to write this series of books – I hope you find them helpful.

For the last few years, I have been working as a doctor in the media alongside my clinical practice. I started by answering medical queries on a consumer health website, which lead to me being asked to write for various magazines and, ultimately, appear on television and radio. In 2013, we celebrated our one hundredth episode of *Embarrassing Bodies*. There have been several more episodes since, and I hope there will be more to come. I am now one of the regular doctors on ITV's *This Morning* and do a weekly Health Hour phone-in on LBC radio. My media work has shown me time and time again that people often leave the consulting room with unanswered questions. Maybe you forgot to ask, or maybe there simply wasn't enough time, and I guess that is the other reason for the Dr Dawn Guides. My aim for these books is to address all those unanswered questions.

Women's health has special meaning for me. For the first ten years of my general practice career, I was the only female partner in a seven-doctor practice, which meant, inevitably, that I saw a lot of women. I have always believed that we enjoy, both socially and professionally, the things that we are good at. I was never going to change the fact that many women, understandably, prefer to see a female doctor for breast-related or gynaecological problems. Let's face it, if you have terrible periods or you want to divorce your husband every four weeks because it is 'that time of the month', at least you know I have had periods and can empathise to a degree with your dilemma! So, I set out to do some extra work in my local gynaecology department working in clinics and on-call. It paid off. I learned a lot about everything related to women's health, and it has been an area of medicine that I have always enjoyed.

My aim in this book is to cover those conditions specific to us girls. As women, we are juggling aspects of our lives today more than ever before and our own health needs can so easily fall to the bottom of a long list. This book will be your one-stop shop for all female health issues. I will explain everything from breast to period problems, incontinence to managing the menopause, and much more. I will tell you what to expect from tests and treatment, how to manage your condition, how to make the most of your appointments and what symptoms not to avoid. I hope you won't need the information in this book, but if you do, I will help make your diagnosis easy to understand and your journey through your treatment as stress free as possible.

1

Breast disease

I have chosen to start with this condition for the simple reason that nothing gets a woman into my GP consulting room faster than a new-found lump in her breast. In fact, the majority of breast lumps are benign. Many don't require a referral to a specialist and, of those that do, nine out of ten lumps turn out to be benign; but breast cancer is the most common cancer in women and one in eight of us will develop the condition at some point in our lives. So the bottom line is that any breast lump needs to be checked out.

Who gets breast cancer?

Being female and getting older are the two biggest factors increasing the risk of developing breast cancer. There are around 50,000 new cases of breast cancer in women in the UK every year – that's approximately one new case diagnosed every ten minutes – compared to about 300 cases a year in men. Three-quarters of all female breast cancers occur in women over 50, but, of course, it's the breast cancers that occur in younger women that hit our headlines – 1 in 20 breast cancers develop in women under the age of 35. Having a first degree relative – a sister, mother or daughter – with the disease increases your risk and in some families we can identify genes that significantly increase the risk of developing the disease, but more of that later. Women who start their periods very young or who have a late menopause are at increased risk because of their higher lifetime exposure to the female hormone oestrogen.

So those are the things you can't do a lot about! What about the things we can influence? Women who don't have children or who start their family late (after age 30) are also at risk, but breast feeding is protective. It is estimated that being overweight is a factor in almost one in ten breast cancer cases, so maintaining a health body mass index (BMI) reduces your risk. Excess alcohol intake and smoking will also increase your risk, so watch these and keep an eye on your diet – a high-fat diet increases the risk of developing breast cancer. X-rays, even in small doses, can also mean you are more likely to develop the disease.

How do we screen for breast cancer?

I'm a great fan of women being what I call **breast aware**. It's your job to know what is normal for you so that you can report any changes, and it is my job to know whether you need further assessment. But before you start feeling, get into the habit of looking at your breasts. This may seem strange at first, but you will notice that your breasts are not totally symmetrical – the only perfectly symmetrical breasts that I see are silicone and, believe me, I have seen a lot of breasts! It is normal for one to be slightly larger than the other, but if the difference in size is changing then your doctor needs to know. Take some time to look at the skin – any new tethering or dimpling needs to be checked out. Then, the easiest way to examine your own breasts is using a soapy hand, in a warm shower or bath, so that you can feel with the flat of your hand: work your way around the breast and into the armpit, as there is a tail of breast tissue that extends up into the armpit. Finally, gently squeeze both nipples to check for any discharge. It is possible to get a milky discharge from the nipple even when not breast feeding but any new discharge needs to be checked out, especially if it is only occurs on one side or is blood stained.

If you are registered with an NHS GP, you will automatically be called sometime after your fiftieth birthday for a mammogram and, when you get that letter, I would urge you to go. You may not relish the idea of having your breasts squeezed in a machine but, believe me, the reassurance of a normal mammogram is worth it, and if you are given bad news, as with all cancers, early diagnosis of breast cancer can make all the difference to a good prognosis.

Once you are on the screening register you will be called every three years until you are 70; the screening programme is soon to be extended to include all women between 47 and 73. If you want to continue to be screened after this age, simply call your local service to arrange it. Some women (those who have a strong family history of breast cancer) will be offered mammography at a younger age.

How is breast cancer diagnosed?

Breast cancer is either picked up at a routine screening mammogram or is diagnosed after a woman has presented to her GP with symptoms; the most common sympton being a painless lump. If a woman presents with a lump that is cause for concern, in the first instance she will almost certainly be offered a mammogram and possibly an ultrasound of her breasts. Ultrasound is particularly useful in pre-menopausal women who have more dense breast tissue. Sometimes a magnetic resonance imaging (MRI) scan will be arranged. What happens after this will depend on what the tests have shown. Some women will undergo a needle biopsy where a sample of breast tissue is removed under local anaesthetic to be viewed under the microscope. Others may have what is called an **excision biopsy**, where the entire lump is removed for analysis. If a biopsy tests positive for cancer, then further tests will be done to check whether the cancer has spread and these can include blood tests, X-rays and scans.

What is the breast cancer gene?

There are several genes that have been identified that are associated with an increased risk of developing breast cancer, and if you have a strong family history of the disease you may be offered genetic testing to look for genes including *BRCA1*, *BRCA2* and *TP53*. If a woman tests positive for *BRCA1* she has an 80–85 per cent chance of developing breast cancer and would be offered prophylactic bilateral mastectomy. This is where both breasts are surgically removed, leaving no breast tissue, which radically reduces the risk of developing breast cancer.

What is staging?

Once a diagnosis of breast cancer is made, the team of doctors and nurses looking after you will want to stage the disease. By this they mean they will work out how big the cancer is and how far it has spread, because this will influence the treatment plan. There are six stages:

- Stage 0 – the cancer is localized and not invasive;
- Stage 1 – the tumour is less than 2 cm in diameter and there is no spread;
- Stage 2 – the tumour is between 2 and 5 cm in diameter or there is spread to the armpit on that side;
- Stage 3a – the tumour is more than 5 cm in diameter and lymph nodes in the armpit are stuck down;
- Stage 3b – when a tumour of any size has spread to the surrounding skin and other lymph nodes;
- Stage 4 – the tumour has spread to other parts of the body such as the bones, liver or brain.

How do we treat breast cancer?

Treatment can include any combination of surgery, chemotherapy, hormonal therapy and radiotherapy. Most breast cancers in the UK are treated with surgical excision of the lump only, avoiding a mastectomy, and radiotherapy, but each decision has to be made according to the stage of the disease and each woman's wishes. If there are multiple tumours or the lump is more than 4 cm in diameter, you will probably be offered a mastectomy and it is important that you have the opportunity to discuss with your surgeon whether you would be suitable for reconstructive surgery at the same time. Some women may be advised against this. Radiotherapy, for example, can hinder wound healing and it may be better to wait until later for reconstruction. Some tumours have hormone receptors and women with this sort of tumour will be offered hormonal therapy.

Benign breast lumps

I have already said that the majority of breast lumps are not cancerous, so what are they? Most commonly they are fibroadenomas or cysts. A fibroadenoma is also sometimes called a breast mouse – it is firm to touch but can be moved around under the skin of the breast. They are most common in younger women aged between 15 and 30. They are not cancerous, so don't need to be removed and one in five will disappear on their own anyway, but women with fibroadenomas have a very slightly increased risk of developing breast cancer. Breast cysts tend to occur in older women aged between 40 and 50, and in about 50 per cent of cases there will be multiple cysts. Cysts are fluid-filled sacks, which can be removed by being aspirated with a needle, but they return in about 10 per cent of cases.

Breast pain

In three-quarters of women presenting with breast pain, the pain is linked to the menstrual cycle and may also be associated with lumpiness in the breast. The symptoms develop on the run up to a period and resolve after the period begins. This sort of breast pain is most common in women in their twenties and is referred to as cyclical breast pain. Non-cyclical breast pain tends to occur in older women and has no link to the menstrual cycle. Cyclical breast pain will resolve of its own accord in about one-third of cases and, for non-cyclical breast pain, in half of women who have it. A well-fitted bra, simple pain killers and anti-inflammatory drugs should be the first port of call for treatment. Changing from the combined contraceptive pill to a non-hormonal form of contraception may help women struggling with cyclical breast pain. If the pain is very localized, it sometimes responds well to an injection of local anaesthetic and steroid. If cyclical breast pain is still causing trouble despite these simple measures then your doctor may suggest various hormone treatments available on prescription.

Nipple discharge

It is not uncommon for women to notice a milky discharge from their nipples during pregnancy or when on the combined contraceptive pill. It can also occur following stimulation of the nipple during foreplay, but there are other causes and it should always be checked out. Some medicines cause nipple discharge, including some blood pressure treatments, antidepressants and an indigestion remedy called cimetidine. If you suspect your medicine could be to blame, don't stop taking it without talking to your doctor first, but it is worth asking if you could try an alternative. Street drugs, such as cannabis, heroine and speed, can all cause nipple discharge and some herbal remedies, including fennel, fenugreek seed, marsh mallow, anise, blessed thistle, nettle, red clover and red raspberry, can also be to blame.

Nipple discharge that is only from one nipple, or that is blood stained, is more of a worry as it could indicate an underlying cancer, particular in women over 45, and needs to be seen urgently. Your doctor will probably want to arrange some blood tests to check your hormones. One in five women with a milky discharge, known as **galactorrhoea**, will have a tumour in the pituitary gland in the brain and will need scans and tests to look into this.

2

Menstrual problems

The average age at which girls start their periods in the UK is 13. This is younger than a century ago, which is probably due to improved nutrition and increasing weight. There are critical weights at which our hormones kick in and, in fact, shut down, which is why very thin athletes and anorexic girls often stop having periods altogether. But starting your periods anywhere between the ages of 8 and 16 is deemed normal – girls who start their periods before the age of 8 should be taken to their GPs, as should those who are yet to see their first period over the age of 16.

What is a normal cycle?

We talk of a normal menstrual cycle as being 28 days long with ovulation occurring in the middle, but anything from 21 days to 35 is considered within normal limits. If you are trying to predict ovulation, it is important to remember that ovulation occurs 14 days *before* the first day of a period, not 14 days *after* a period. Of course, if your cycle is 28 days, these are one and the same but if you have a regular 21-day cycle, for example, your fertile time (when you ovulate) will be 14 days before your period – this is just 7 days after Day 1 of your previous period (Day 1 is the first day of bleeding). Worth bearing in mind if you are timing sex to either avoid your fertile time or to conceive!

As your period starts a gland in your brain, called the pituitary gland, is already producing a hormone called follicle stimulating hormone (FSH) that, as it's name suggests, stimulates the development of follicles in your ovary. As a follicle matures it produces oestrogen and, as oestrogen levels rise, messages are fed back to the brain to stop producing FSH. Once oestrogen levels are high enough, the pituitary produces a second hormone, luteinizing hormone. This surge of luteinizing hormone is what triggers ovulation, which occurs within about 36 hours. An egg is released from the ovary and travels along the fallopian tube to the womb, where the lining has thickened ready to nurture a fertilized egg and develop a pregnancy. If pregnancy does not occur, that thickened lining is shed and this is what we recognize as a period. And then the cycle starts all over again.

What is normal and what is heavy menstrual bleeding?

All women vary and each individual will notice differences in their periods from time to time. Average blood loss has been calculated though and is thought to be around 40 ml per period. That is just eight teaspoons over the average of five or six days that a woman bleeds. I find that women are often surprised by how little that is. It feels a lot more, doesn't it? But you only have to see a child with a nose bleed to appreciate that a small amount of blood can go a long way.

Heavy periods or menorrhagia, from the Greek *men* (month) and *rhegynai* (to rush out), are one of the most common complaints about periods that GPs hear. Strictly speaking, the definition of menorrhagia is a blood loss of more than 16 teaspoons (80 ml) per cycle; this level of blood loss will almost certainly result in anaemia so needs to be treated. But who measures their menstrual loss? Those using a moon cup to collect menstrual blood, rather than pads or tampons, may have a more accurate idea but as far as I am concerned if your periods are stopping you from carrying on your normal daily life then you should see your GP as there are plenty of things we can do to help. And of course what is acceptable to one woman will be totally unacceptable to another for lots of different reasons. It may be related to what you are used to, or to your mother's and sister's experiences. Some women are more robust than others and, of course, what you have to do in your day will have an influence too. If you work from home and don't have to go out, heavy periods are much less likely to cause you problems than if you are having to travel long distances or spend hours in meetings unable to get to a loo. However, passing clots and flooding are generally accepted as heavy periods and are not something you have to put up with.

What will my doctor do about my heavy periods?

Your GP will want to take a detailed medical history from you, so before you make the appointment try to jot down how long this has been a problem, how many days you bleed for and how frequently, and if you can give him or her an idea of how often you are changing pads or tampons that will be helpful too. If it is normal for you to need to use pads and tampons together you are almost certainly putting up with something you shouldn't be!

Your GP will want to examine your cervix to check for polyps, which can cause heavy bleeding, and to do an internal examination to check the size of the uterus. If the uterus is enlarged, your doctor will arrange an ultrasound. By far the most common cause of an enlarged uterus (apart from pregnancy, when of course your periods will have stopped!) is fibroids. Fibroids are very common – around half of all women aged 50 will have fibroids. They often don't cause any trouble at all and tend to shrink after the menopause, but if they do cause problems, they are most likely to lead to heavy menstrual bleeding. Often we don't find a specific cause, which is known as **dysfunctional uterine bleeding**. Your doctor will also arrange a blood test to check your heavy bleeding hasn't left you anaemic, and if he or she is concerned that you have a problem with your thyroid,which can be linked to heavy periods, or have a more generalized problem with easy bleeding your doctor may do blood tests for these conditions too.

What treatments are available for heavy periods?

The first line of treatment is usually something called an intra-uterine system, which is like a contraceptive coil but which secretes tiny amounts of hormone into the lining of the womb to reduce blood flow. It is very effective and can be fitted by your GP. The amount of hormone that is released into your system is the same as taking two mini pills a week. If this is not suitable for you, your doctor may suggest some anti-inflammatory-type pills on prescription that can reduce blood flow by between 25 and 50 per cent. They are only taken around the time of bleeding and are non-hormonal. Alternatively, you could try the combined contraceptive pill which reduces blood flow by around a half or you could try taking progestogens.

If none of these measures work, you may be referred for an endometrial ablation. This is a day-case procedure done under anaesthetic where the lining of the womb is removed but the womb itself is left in place. It is so effective that the number of hysterectomies that are performed each year in the UK has fallen dramatically since this technique was developed. Other options are to block the artery supplying the womb, a procedure known as **uterine artery embolization**, to remove the muscle of the womb (myomectomy) or, as a last resort, to perform a full hysterectomy and remove the entire womb. In other words, there are lots of different treatment options open to you. I have met too many women who have put up with heavy periods for too long because they thought it was a hysterectomy or nothing and they didn't want such a major operation. So if you are struggling, don't put up with it anymore – make that appointment.

Painful periods (dysmenorrhoea)

Most of us will get some pain with our periods but around one in ten women suffer with so much pain that their periods prevent them getting on with their day to day life. Severe pain with periods is more common in younger women and the good news is that things often improve as we get older. There isn't usually any specific cause but if painful periods start in your 30s or 40s then this could be linked to a problem in the pelvis. This is called **secondary dysmenorrhoea**. Let's deal with the far more common form, primary dysmenorrhoea, first.

Primary dysmenorrhoea

We don't really know why this affects some women and not others. There are a couple of theories though – one is that the chemicals called prostaglandins, which build up in the lining of the womb to help it to contract and shed, are present in higher concentrations in some women; another is that some women are simply more sensitive to their effects. Period pain, just like labour pain, can be felt in the lower tummy, in the thighs and/or lower back. It usually starts a day or so before the bleeding begins and can last for a few days.

What can my doctor do?

Your GP will listen to your story and, unless there are specific things that make your doctor suspect a secondary cause, an examination probably won't be necessary. There are various things your doctor may advise, depending on the severity of your symptoms. Simple measures like holding a hot water bottle against your tummy or taking paracetamol may suffice for relatively mild symptoms, but women struggling with more severe symptoms may need to take anti-inflammatory drugs. Some, such as ibuprofen, you can buy over the counter at the pharmacy but others will need a prescription from your GP. Taking the combined contraceptive pill tends to lighten periods and make them less painful and there are other progestogen contraceptives that may help if you can't take oestrogen. The intra-uterine system used to lighten (or, in many women, stop) periods is another option. I am often asked about more natural remedies, such as herbal or dietary supplements. The jury is out on these – there is no good evidence that they are effective so my feeling is that more work needs to be done to assess their role before we recommend them.

What is secondary dysmenorrhoea?

Secondary dysmenorrhoea is when periods suddenly become painful having not been a problem before. It is normal for the first few periods that a girl has to be painless and then to become more painful as the cycles regulate, but if an older woman starts having problems this is called **secondary amenorrhoea**. If the pain is associated with a change in bleeding pattern, bleeding between periods, a vaginal discharge or pain during sex, your GP will want to investigate further with a pelvic examination and possibly other tests, such an ultrasound of your womb or using a telescope called a laparoscope to look around the outside of your womb through a small cut near your tummy button, or using a hysteroscope to look inside the womb through your cervix. From there, the treatment will depend on what the tests reveal (see Chapters 7 and 9).

Absent periods (amenorrhoea)

Just like dysmenorrhoea, amenorrhoea can be primary, where the periods never start, or secondary, for women whose periods were normal but have now stopped. If periods haven't started by the age of 16, your doctor may want to do some tests to look into possible causes.

What causes primary amenorrhoea?

Some girls may have been born without a womb, which, of course, is often only noticed when periods don't start and an ultrasound confirms its absence. It is also possible to be born with a womb which has no passage to the outside. In this case girls may notice period-type pains each month but no bleeding. If periods never start and there are no other signs of puberty, such as breast development and pubic hair, this could be caused by a hormonal problem or a rare syndrome, so your GP will want to arrange some tests.

What causes secondary amenorrhoea?

By far and away the most common cause of secondary amenorrhoea is pregnancy and, since no form of contraception is 100 per cent effective, if your periods suddenly stop a pregnancy test should be your first port of call! The second is probably the menopause and while the average age for the menopause in the UK is approximately 51, it is possible to go through the change much earlier. A menopause before 40 is described as a premature menopause and I have met women in their twenties who are going through 'the change'. Your GP will be able run blood tests for this.

Other causes include breast feeding and some forms of progesterone-only contraception, such as the injection, the implant and the intra-uterine system. It is also relatively common to find that there is a delay in starting periods after stopping the combined contraceptive pill. Periods usually resume within six months though, and if they don't, other possibilities should be checked out. Significant weight loss will also stop periods as nature considers very thin women to be unable to carry a healthy pregnancy so shuts down their hormones, which is why anorexic girls and some very thin athletes stop their periods. Polycystic ovaries (see Chapter 10) are another common cause. There are other rare causes, such as severe narrowing of the neck of the womb and diseases that affect the pituitary gland that produces the hormones to drive the ovaries.

What about abnormal menstrual bleeding?

Bleeding that occurs after sex (post-coital bleeding), between periods (inter-menstrual bleeding) and bleeding after a woman has gone through the menopause (post-menopausal bleeding) should always be reported to your doctor.

Post-coital bleeding

The most common cause of this is an erosion on the cervix. These are particularly common in women taking the combined contraceptive pill and don't usually cause any problems, but if they do, bleeding after sex is a common one. Your doctor will be able to see if you have an erosion with a speculum examination, just like when you have a smear. If the problem persists, your cervix can be painted with a special paint to dry up the erosion. You may need more than one treatment. Polyps in the cervical canal or in the womb can also cause post-coital bleeding. Gynaecological cancers, such as cancer of the vagina, cervix or womb, can also cause these symptoms, which is why it is so important not to ignore them.

Inter-menstrual bleeding

In a very small number of women bleeding mid cycle is just a sign of ovulation but this really is only one or two in every hundred, and far more commonly inter-menstrual bleeding is down to missed contraceptive pills or a sexually transmitted infection. In fact unless there is an obvious cause such as missed pills, I assume that inter-menstrual bleeding is due to chlamydia or gonorrhoea until proved otherwise, and it is important that these infections are tested for. Fibroids and gynaecological cancers can also cause inter-menstrual bleeding, but if there is any suggestion that this is the case, your GP will arrange the necessary tests.

Post-menopausal bleeding

Post-menopausal bleeding is defined as bleeding that occurs 12 or more months after the menopause and it should always be looked into. Most cases will not be anything to be worried about but, just like inter-menstrual bleeding being chlamydia until proved otherwise, uterine cancer must always be excluded in any woman with post-menopausal bleeding. Your GP will test for this with an ultrasound test to check out the thickness of the uterine lining and an endometrial biopsy. This can be done by your doctor and involves a tiny instrument being inserted through the cervix to take a sample of cells from the womb lining for analysis under a microscope. I have done literally hundreds of these and had very, very few positive results but it is always better to be safe than sorry.

Toxic shock syndrome

Toxic shock syndrome is one of those conditions that just about every menstruating woman has heard of, and is terrified of, but in fact in all my years of practice I have only ever seen one case. In contrast, I have removed hundreds of forgotten tampons which have been left for days, and sometimes even weeks. Toxic shock syndrome is thankfully rare and, due to developments in tampon manufacture, is becoming more so, but it is a life-threatening condition so one we must consider. It presents with a high fever and there may be an associated red rash all over the body. It can cause sickness and diarrhoea, and muscle aches. These sort of symptoms can easily be put down to food poisoning, or tummy upsets, so always just think about whether you could have left a tampon inside. If toxic shock syndrome is left undiagnosed a patient can rapidly deteriorate, becoming confused and developing kidney and liver failure. High dose antibiotics, given promptly, will treat the condition but delay could be fatal: 5–15 per cent of people who develop toxic shock syndrome will not survive.

3

Pre-menstrual syndrome

Pre-menstrual syndrome (PMS) is thought to affect at least 1 in 20 women and, I suspect, many more because a lot of women don't seek help. The symptoms vary between different women and can vary from cycle to cycle in the same woman, but the defining factor for diagnosis is a clear story that symptoms build in the run up to a period and are then relieved when the period starts. If your symptoms persist throughout your cycle then it is not PMS and you and your doctor should think again about the diagnosis. Typically symptoms of PMS worsen about six days before a period and peak a couple of days before bleeding starts. Symptoms should improve significantly within a few days of the period starting. Keeping a symptom diary is the best way to confirm whether or not your symptoms could be attributed to PMS.

What are the symptoms of PMS?

The most common symptoms are irritability, frustration and upset. I often see women in surgery who tell me that they want to divorce their husbands in the run up to their period, that they are screaming at the kids and not coping with demands at work, but as soon as the period starts their world is a different place. The crazy thing is that once you have identified that the symptoms are down to PMS, you would think that you could talk yourself out of the upset but it doesn't work that way. In fact pointing out to a premenstrual woman that she is being a little irrational is tantamount to waving the proverbial red rag to a bull! There may also be physical symptoms such as breast pain, bloating and fluid retention, and because of the emotional upset these physical symptoms may be less well tolerated than normal.

Who gets PMS?

Any woman can suffer with PMS and it can start at any time in a woman's reproductive life. Interestingly, if your Mum suffered then you are more likely to. We don't know why, but women who smoke are more likely to develop PMS and women with a poor diet and who don't exercise are also at increased risk. Women who underachieve academically are more likely to experience premenstrual symptoms.

How is PMS treated?

Recognizing that your symptoms are PMS is the first step to improving things for yourself. Some simple lifestyle changes may make all the difference so try cutting out excess sugar and swap to eating small quantities of complex carbohydrates every two to three hours. Examples of complex carbohydrates are beans, nuts, lentils, oats and wholemeal grains, and cereals. Cutting down on saturated fat and caffeine in your diet and investing in a good support bra may help reduce breast pain, and support stockings will help relieve aching legs. If fluid retention is an issue for you, watch your salt intake. Try not to add salt to your food. It may taste a little bland at first, but your taste buds adapt surprisingly quickly and within a couple of weeks you will have adjusted. Regular exercise and getting out in natural daylight will improve your mood and help you relax. Try to plan ahead. Look at your diary and wherever possible try to avoid high pressure meetings and deadlines the week before a period is due. Don't fill up your diary on the run up to a period, but be realistic about how you are going to feel. There is nothing wrong with explaining to friends and family that you know you won't need that extra pressure at that time.

What can my doctor do?

Lots! So don't suffer in silence. The most effective treatment is one of the newer class of antidepressants called **selective serotonin reuptake inhibitors**. I find many women shy away from taking these drugs but those that are willing to try them find they are life changing, and I am sure they have saved many a marriage. Contrary to popular belief they are not addictive. If you really don't want to go down that route, a lot of my patients tell me they have found St John's Wort helpful. It is a herbal remedy so doesn't have the same strict licensing criteria as a medicine, but if you buy some that has a patient information leaflet in the packaging, then that particular product has been licensed voluntarily and you know you are getting what it says on the packaging. Alternatively, you could try the combined contraceptive pill. Taking three packs back to back with no breaks, so that you only have four bleeds a year, has been shown to reduce frequency of symptoms. In extreme cases, having injections to switch off your hormones and then replacing them with a regulated dose of hormone is an option.

Every few months I meet a woman who is so fed up with her PMS that she just wants 'it all out'. Having a hysterectomy is a pretty drastic measure and should be considered a last resort. You need to be absolutely certain that your symptoms are premenstrual, and that you have completed your family. It is an option but there is no going back so I like to try the injections first to make sure that switching off your ovaries really will make things better and you need to be very clear about the long-term implications of going through a surgical menopause at a young age (see Chapter 4).

4

Menopause

Baby girls are born with a finite number of follicles in their ovaries. These will start developing at puberty and once periods are established will continue to mature each month until they run out and then the menopause occurs. The run up to the menopause is often associated with erratic cycles and other symptoms and, strictly speaking, this stage should be referred to as the perimenopause or climacteric. The menopause itself can actually only be diagnosed with certainty a year after periods stop. The average age for the menopause in the UK is 51, but it can occur any time between 40 and 58. A menopause that occurs before the age of 45 is called an **early menopause**, and one that happens to a woman under 40 is referred to as a **premature menopause**. The greater your BMI, the later your menopause is likely to be, while smokers may experience an earlier menopause. If your Mum had an early menopause, you are more likely to have one too and it may occur even earlier than hers, which is worth bearing in mind if your Mum had a premature menopause. I have met a small number of women who had a family history like that, who weren't warned and sadly missed out on the opportunity to have a family because the menopause came much earlier than they were expecting. The earlier you start your periods the more quickly you will go through your follicles, but being on the combined contraceptive pill prevents the maturation of follicles so will give you extra time before your menopause. By the same reckoning, the more pregnancies you have, the later your menopause will be.

What are the symptoms of the menopause?

Each woman's experience of the menopause is very individual. Eight out of ten women will get some of the symptoms mentioned below, which means that two out of ten lucky ladies will simply stop their periods without other associated symptoms. Of those that have symptoms, some will be mild and others will really struggle. I am often asked how long the flushes and so on will last and, sadly I'm afraid, that is crystal ball territory – some women will have problems for a few months, others struggle for several years. Only about one in ten women just stop their periods suddenly. Much more commonly, periods become erratic on the run up to the menopause. Some women find their periods become more frequent and sometimes heavier, while others report longer cycles and, on average, this time of less predictable cycles can last around four years.

I think the most common symptoms that bring women into my surgery are hot flushes, night sweats and mood swings. We all experience tiny fluctuations in body temperature several times a day and it is something that we are totally unaware of. But in the perimenopausal woman, there is a heightened sensitivity to these minute temperature differences and this is what causes the sweats and flushes. Even drinking a hot drink can trigger a flush. Some women will have the occasional flush, whereas others can experience flushes several times an hour; and while these symptoms generally last anything from a few months to up to seven years, I have met some ladies who are still struggling a decade on.

The mood swings also cause a great deal of distress. I have some ladies who tell me that without hormone replacement therapy they would be divorced, friendless and jobless! The menopause can wreak havoc with concentration and confidence. I have met women who have run high-powered businesses and who have fallen apart at the menopause because they can't even decide which knickers to put on in the morning!

Women often tell me that their memory is shocking and that they feel anxious or nervous a lot of the time. Some get depressed, and many go off sex altogether. The lack of libido can be linked to feelings of low self-esteem and realizations of getting older, but it may also be because of vaginal dryness making sex uncomfortable. Sadly, while most women (and men for that matter) are fully aware that the menopause can be associated with flushes and mood swings, very few seem to know that vaginal dryness is a very common menopausal symptom. As oestrogen levels fall, the tissues around the vagina become thinner and drier, which can cause sex to be uncomfortable and may cause symptoms of cystitis. This is something you don't need to put up with even if you don't want hormone replacement therapy (HRT). I can't tell you how many times I have done a smear on a perimenopausal woman and noticed the vaginal skin looks a little inflamed. When I then ask about sex, I am usually given one of two replies, either 'Sex? What's that?' or 'My husband is very patient and we don't do it very often anymore'. If you are both happy with a less active sex life then that is fine, but if it is having a detrimental effect on your relationship then some oestrogen pessaries or cream that is used in the vagina can make a real difference.

We are all too politically correct to use such terms as **middle-aged spread** today, but just because we don't talk about it, it doesn't mean it doesn't happen! I'm afraid we are more likely to put down fat around our middles after the menopause. Other less well-known symptoms include thinning hair, thinning of the skin, brittle nails and generalized aches and pains.

Can a blood test confirm the menopause?

I think I am probably asked this question most weeks but, sadly, blood tests in the perimenopause are notoriously unreliable. Once periods have stopped and the menopause is obvious, levels of the hormone that drives our ovaries, follicle stimulating hormone or FSH, rise as the brain desperately tries to get our failing ovaries to do their thing. But in the perimenopause, FSH levels fluctuate all over the place. As far as I am concerned, if a woman is the right age and she has classic menopausal symptoms then it doesn't matter what her FSH level is, she is perimenopausal until proved otherwise!

Can lifestyle affect menopausal symptoms?

Maintaining a healthy weight and taking regular exercise will not only help menopausal symptoms, but will also reduce the risk of osteoporosis (see the section in this chapter about the long-term benefits of HRT). You should also ensure that your diet contains at least 1500 mg of calcium a day to help protect your bones.

Stopping smoking and only drinking the recommended amount of alcohol will also help. You need to be honest about your alcohol intake. The recommended limit for women is 14 units a week, which is surprisingly little. You can calculate your intake by looking at the percentage alcohol in the drink you are drinking. The percentage alcohol shows you the number of units in a litre of that drink; so, for wine, a 75 cl bottle is three-quarters of a litre (75 cl = 750 ml; 1 litre = 1000 ml), so if the wine contains 12 per cent alcohol, the number of units in the bottle is three-quarters of 12 = 9 units. If you are pouring a glass at home it is likely to be a 250 ml glass and that will contain three units!

Hormone replacement therapy

It's not that long ago that I could barely complete a surgery without seeing a menopausal woman asking for HRT. Today I see only a few, and that's a shame. All those women who would have been in my consulting room a few years ago are still struggling; they have just been put off by scary headlines. HRT is undoubtedly the most effective way to treat menopausal symptoms and the decision on whether or not to take it will depend on the severity of each individual woman's symptoms and her personal medical history. It's certainly worth having the conversation with your doctor.

HRT comes in the form of tablets, patches, gels, a ring that is inserted into the vagina, and there is even a nasal spray. If you choose to start HRT, your doctor will explain the different forms to you and which one you choose will mostly be down to personal preference, although there are some specific guidelines. Most women will take a combination of oestrogen and progesterone. We need the oestrogen to combat the menopausal symptoms, but if you take oestrogen alone without the protection of progesterone there is an increased risk of developing cancer of the womb. If you have had a hysterectomy, your doctor will suggest a form of oestrogen-only HRT. If you are still having periods, your doctor will advise you to take a form of cyclical combined HRT where you take oestrogen only for the first part of a cycle and then a combination of oestrogen and progesterone for the second half, which will be followed by a bleed. This is not a period in the true sense because you will not have ovulated but it resembles the normal menstrual cycle. There is also the option of having a three-monthly cyclical HRT where you only bleed every three months. If you start HRT a year or more after your last natural period, you will be directed towards a continuous combined form of HRT where you take both hormones every day and you should not, therefore, have any bleeding.

How quickly will HRT work?

HRT is extremely effective at treating menopausal symptoms. Hot flushes and night sweats often start to improve within four weeks, but can take up to three months to respond. The changes in the vagina can take a little longer and improvement can take up to a year. Sometimes I prescribe oestrogen pessaries or vaginal cream as well as conventional HRT to help with this.

What about the long-term benefits of HRT?

There is no doubt that women who take HRT have a reduced risk of developing osteoporosis and recent evidence has shown that women under 60 taking HRT are less likely to experience cardiovascular disease. Interestingly, though, the exact opposite is true in women over the age of 60 taking HRT.

What are the risks associated with HRT?

You are more likely to develop a blood clot if you are on HRT tablets, particularly if you are overweight or smoke. Interestingly, this is not the case if you take HRT in patch form. There is an increased risk of stroke or heart disease in women over the age of 60 taking HRT. There is a small increased risk of developing breast cancer if you take HRT, and I mean *small* – taking HRT equates to one extra case of breast cancer per thousand women each year, and five years after stopping HRT your risk is the same as if you had never taken it. There is also a very small increased risk of ovarian cancer in women taking HRT. If you are at high risk of developing any of these conditions because of your lifestyle or your family or medical history, your doctor may advise you against HRT.

Does HRT cause weight gain?

I can't tell you how often women have decided against HRT because they are concerned about possible weight gain. Unfortunately, the menopause is often associated with putting on a few extra pounds, usually around the midriff, and so often women come back to me a few months after they have started HRT having gained a few pounds, which, of course they have blamed on HRT. However, there is no evidence that HRT will cause you to put on a significant amount of weight.

Will I get recurrent menopausal symptoms when I stop HRT?

Some women get menopausal symptoms when they come off HRT, but we can reduce the severity and duration of these symptoms by weaning down slowly – so don't just decide to stop your HRT. Make sure you discuss the best way to do this with your doctor.

What about contraception when I'm taking HRT?

Don't forget, HRT is not a contraceptive and whether you choose to take it or not you will need to use contraception for a year after your last natural period if that occurs after the age of 50. If your last natural period occurs under the age of 50 you will need contraception for two years.

What are the alternatives to HRT?

Lots of women look for relief in the form of herbal remedies, one of the most popular being phytoestrogens, which are naturally occurring oestrogen-like substances found in plants and foods such as soya. I am told that there is no direct translation of the term *hot flush* in the Japanese language and this is thought to be because Japanese women don't suffer like we do, the theory being that their diet is naturally rich in soya. Phytoestrogens are effective at relieving hot flushes and sweats, but I am a firm believer that if anything is good enough to do some good then it could also have the same negative effects as conventional medicines that do the same job. So, if your doctor advises against taking oestrogen you should probably avoid these too. There are also some non-hormonal prescription medicines that may help, including the selective serotonin reuptake inhibitors and an old-fashioned blood pressure treatment called clonidine.

Should I have a DEXA scan?

A DEXA scan is a special type of X-ray which is used to assess bone density. We know that our bones start to thin after the menopause and if you have had an early menopause (under the age of 45), or if you are post-menopausal and smoke or drink heavily, or have a BMI under 21, or a strong family history of osteoporosis, your GP may recommend that you have a DEXA scan. You will also be advised to have a DEXA scan if you experience a fracture after a relatively minor injury.

5

Cystitis

Cystitis simply means inflammation of the bladder lining. It may be caused by infection from bacteria, viruses or fungi, but can also be due to irritation from chemicals. It surprises many people when they hear that urine is actually sterile and the presence of any bugs is abnormal. The problem can be deciding whether the presence of bacteria in urine is due to contamination by bacteria from the surrounding skin or whether there is a bladder infection present; this decision is generally made on the grounds of concentration – the greater the number of bacteria, the more significant their presence is likely to be.

What are the symptoms of cystitis and how is it treated?

Around one in five women will have a urinary tract infection in their lifetimes and will experience the classic symptoms of needing to go to the loo urgently, only to find there is very little urine to pass and what does come out stings and burns. Some will also experience pain in the lower abdomen. If you see your doctor with these symptoms, he or she will almost certainly want to dipstick test your urine looking for the presence of white blood cells (leucocytes) and nitrites. If this test is positive, then it is almost certain that there is a bacterial infection requiring treatment. In some women, such as those who are pregnant, have diabetes, or who are known to have abnormalities in the urinary tract, it is usual to send the sample to the lab for further analysis, but, in most cases, the presence of leucocytes and nitrites is enough to warrant a prescription for antibiotics. In some areas of the country there has been growing bacterial resistance to the commonly used antibiotics, but your doctor will know which are likely to be most effective. Strains of the bacteria *E. coli* cause 85 per cent of all urinary tract infections; these bugs are normally found in the gut. The reason us girls are more prone to urinary infections than men is very simple – the bugs can travel up our relatively short urethras (the urethra is the tube linking the bladder to the outside world) much more easily than they can in men.

Why are pregnant women treated differently?

Bacteria thrive when the acidity of the urine changes and this occurs more often in pregnant women. That can mean that the bacteria multiply much more quickly and can cause infection before the symptoms of cystitis develop. In addition, hormonal changes in pregnancy mean that the smooth muscle in the urethral wall relaxes more easily meaning the bacteria have easier access. Undiagnosed urinary tract infection in pregnant women can be associated with premature labour or babies that are smaller than they should be, which is one of the reasons why doctor and midwives seem to become obsessed with your urine when you are pregnant.

What about cystitis in diabetics?

Diabetic women are 40 times more likely to have bacteria in their urine that don't cause symptoms than non-diabetic women, and they are also more prone to unusual infections with fungi. This is because diabetics, unless they have perfect diabetic control, will often have glucose in their urine which acts as the perfect feeding environment for bugs.

What about cystitis in post-menopausal women?

After the menopause the pH of the vagina becomes slightly more alkaline. This means that in post-menopausal women, bacteria can proliferate more effectively causing more urinary tract infections. The dryness in the vagina associated with menopausal change can also cause symptoms mimicking cystitis, and oestrogen cream or pessaries used in the vagina can help restore the normal pH, thereby reducing the likelihood of infection, and relieve symptoms.

What about recurrent cystitis infections?

Some women are plagued with recurrent infections and if this is you, your doctor will probably want to do some tests to check out your urinary tract. An ultrasound test will show if there is a stone somewhere in your urinary system, or other blockage, and if you persistently have blood in your urine on dip testing, you may be referred for a cystoscopy – a look into the bladder under anaesthetic to check there is nothing else going on. In the vast majority of cases, no specific cause is found for recurrent infections. Some women will require low-dose daily antibiotics for several weeks or even months.

How can I help myself if I develop cystitis?

If it hurts to wee, it can be tempting to avoid drinking too much fluid in an attempt to reduce the amount of urine you produce, but actually this is likely to make things worse. Concentrated urine will irritate the bladder lining more, so try to drink plenty – aiming for your urine to be straw coloured, not darker. Avoid fizzy drinks, caffeine and alcohol as all of these can cause bladder irritation in their own right. As can nicotine from cigarettes – so if you need another reason to cut out the ciggies here it is!

Cranberry juice has long been recommended as a self-help treatment for cystitis, and while studies disagree on just how effective it is, there is science behind why it should work. *E. coli* have little hooks that they use to cling onto naturally occurring sugars in the bladder wall. Cranberry juice is rich in these sugars so the theory is that the bugs will let go of the bladder wall, cling on to sugars in the urine instead and be emptied from the bladder when you wee. And, contrary to popular belief, you don't have to take the cranberries as juice, they can be eaten as fruit or taken in tablet form. It won't work for everyone, but I think it is worth a try.

What is honeymoon cystitis?

Some women suffer recurrent symptoms of cystitis following intercourse. This is more common if sex is particularly vigorous or if there is little in the way of foreplay. It is more common in women using the diaphragm as a form of contraception; it isn't clear whether this is because the positioning of the diaphragm itself alters the angle of the bladder neck or whether the spermicidal cream or jelly that is used with this form of contraception alters the vaginal pH. I suspect it is a bit of both. It may not be the most romantic thing in the world but, if you do suffer with honeymoon cystitis, try to get into the habit of emptying the bladder immediately after intercourse so that any bacteria that have hitched a ride on the penis are flushed out before they get a chance to proliferate. If you still have problems, speak to your GP as sometimes a single dose antibiotic after intercourse is all that is required to solve this problem.

What is the urethral syndrome?

In around half of women who develop symptoms of cystitis there is no significant bacterial growth. This can be a cause of huge frustration to both the woman and her doctor. In this instance it is important to check for chlamydia infection. However, there is also no doubt that, despite a supposed clear urine test, some women do seem to respond to antibiotics and this may be because the urine sample was taken before the bacterial load had reached a concentration deemed to be *positive*. Alternatively, it could be that in an attempt to flush the bugs out a woman has drunk copious amounts of fluid and, therefore, reduced the concentration of bacteria in, what is by now, her very dilute urine.

6

Incontinence

Incontinence is leaking of urine – it doesn't have to be emptying your whole bladder involuntarily – and there are several different types. It's difficult to know just how common it is because so many women suffer, often for years, in silence. We do know that incontinence is two to three times more common in women than in men. Current estimates suggest that there are at least 3.5 million women in the UK today struggling with incontinence – and given that less than half of all people suffering with moderate or even severe incontinence actually seek help, I am sure that is a gross underestimate. It's certainly one of those conditions that is usually only mentioned if I ask about it directly, or with a hand on the door handle as the patient is leaving the consulting room. That's always difficult because the chances are if you only mention it as you are leaving, then your consultation time has almost certainly run out. At that point your doctor has one of two options – to invite you back in to discuss it in more depth and risk running late, or to ask you to rebook to discuss it another time. The problem with the latter is that you may never pluck up the courage to come back. It seems that urine is the last taboo. People are much more relaxed today talking about their sex lives and periods, but not about urine. I hope that knowing you are not on your own and that there are so many treatment options, which I will cover in this chapter, that you will be able to jump straight in and make the most of your appointment by talking about any continence problems you have right from the start.

What are the different types of incontinence?

- *Stress incontinence* Urine leaks when pressure is put on the bladder by, for example coughing, sneezing or laughing.
- *Urge incontinence or overactive bladder* This is when the bladder is over sensitive and contracts with very little or no warning.
- *Mixed incontinence* A mixture of the two conditions above.
- *Overflow incontinence* This is usually due to chronic obstruction to the outflow of urine from the bladder. This is the one form that is more common in men and is caused by enlargement of the prostate.

How do you distinguish between the types of incontinence?

Your doctor will want to take a very detailed medical history from you about when you have symptoms, so try to think about this before your appointment as sometimes it can be very obvious from the story alone just which type of problem you have. Your doctor may want to examine you to assess the muscles of your pelvic floor. The tests that he will arrange from there will depend on your individual story: an ultrasound to check if urine remains in the bladder after having a wee can be useful; some women will need **urodynamic studies**, where we look at exactly what happens in your bladder when you wee to decide where the problem is. These studies are not done routinely, but, if your specialist is considering surgery, he or she will probably want to arrange these first to ensure that the correct operation is being done.

Stress incontinence

Stress incontinence is particularly common in women who have had children, especially if they have had multiple pregnancies, big babies and rapid deliveries, which stretch the muscles of the pelvic floor. It is also more common in over-weight people simply because of the pressure that the excess weight puts on the bladder.

The first line of treatment is pelvic floor exercises. It is important that you are taught how to do these properly as I have met lots of women in my time who have been religiously doing their pelvic floor exercises but doing them wrongly which means that if anything they have been straining the muscles and making things worse. A nurse specialist, or physiotherapist who specialises in the pelvic floor, is the best person to show you, but basically you are aiming to replicate the feeling that you would have if you tried to stop the flow of urine midstream. You need to do eight to ten short contractions at least three times a day, followed by some longer contractions where you try to hold that feeling for ten seconds. If done correctly pelvic floor exercises can cure stress incontinence in three-quarters of women. If the muscles have been badly stretched, you may not be able to feel when you are doing it correctly, in which case your therapist may suggest you start with little devices that stimulate the muscles for you so that you get to recognize the sensation you are trying to achieve. There is also medication on prescription which can help and, if you are still struggling, your gynaecologist may recommend surgery. The exact procedure will depend on the severity of your symptoms, the results of your tests and your own wishes. It could be anything from plumping agents injected around the neck of the bladder to help support it, to tapes which can be fitted under local anaesthetic to hitch up the bladder, or more major surgery to repair weakened muscles.

Overactive bladder

For most people the urge to have a wee can be present for half an hour or more before it becomes uncomfortable, and even then it can generally be put off until you can find a toilet. If you have an overactive bladder that urge can come suddenly and needs to be acted on immediately otherwise you leak urine and often the leaks associated with overactive bladder (OAB) are of greater volume than those seen in stress incontinence. Sufferers may need to go to the toilet frequently throughout the day and often several times at night. One in six of us have the condition to a degree, but of those with this condition, around a third will experience episodes of incontinence along with the problems of urgency and frequency.

We don't really know why it happens but there are several things you can do for yourself to improve your symptoms. To start with you need to try to retrain your bladder. In a healthy bladder, an individual will start to get the sensation that they may need the toilet when the bladder is about half full. In OAB that sensation might appear when there are really very small volumes of urine in the bladder. The first thing to do is to make a note of how often you are going to the toilet, and then try to stretch the interval between visits. In the early stages this may only be by a few minutes but gradually your bladder will learn it can cope for longer intervals between emptying.

Stress makes the symptoms of OAB worse so try not to worry about it too much – easier said than done, I know. Nicotine, alcohol, caffeine and fizzy drinks can all irritate an OAB so cut these out altogether if you can, but try to drink normal quantities of fluid. It can be tempting to cut right back on fluid intake in a bid to reduce the amount of urine you produce and, therefore, the frequency of needing the toilet but you could actually make things worse. Concentrated urine can irritate an OAB, so aim for your urine to be straw coloured and make sure you know where the nearest toilet is – worrying that you don't know where it is will only make your symptoms worse. How often we wee depends on how much we drink of course, but on average it is normal to go about five or six times a day passing up to 2 litres a day. OAB sufferers may be going much more frequently and passing tiny volumes, but with the right help this can be reversed. Your GP can prescribe medication to help, which can be used alongside bladder training. You may need to take the medication for a few months and then try coming off it, but some people will need to persevere for longer. Pelvic floor exercises improve symptoms and, in extreme cases, specialists can inject the bladder with botulinum toxin to reduce the contraction in the bladder wall. There are also techniques to stimulate the sacral nerve, and sometimes a piece of bowel wall is used to enlarge the physical size of the bladder. This procedure is called **augmentation cystoplasty**.

7

Chronic pelvic pain

Chronic pelvic pain is a miserable condition, and I have seen it wreck lives and relationships. There are a number of different causes and it can take a long while to reach a diagnosis. If you have chronic pelvic pain, it is worth spending some time thinking about your symptoms before you visit your doctor so that you can give as clear a story as possible of how it affects you. Ask yourself the simple questions below and jot down your answers.

- Where do you feel the pain?
- Does it spread anywhere else?
- What makes it worse or better?
- Is it linked to your periods and, if so, how?
- Is it linked to intercourse?
- Do you have any associated vaginal discharge?
- Are there any urinary symptoms?
- Are there any bowel symptoms?

What causes chronic pelvic pain?

Pelvic pain can be due to a number of different conditions and your description of your pain will help your doctor to narrow down the possible causes for you, which is why it is important to spend some time thinking about the nature of your pain.

Endometriosis
Pelvic pain caused by endometriosis characteristically starts a couple of days before a period starts and lasts throughout the period. It is felt in the lower abdomen and can go through

to the back or radiate down to the thighs. Endometriosis can also be associated with pain on intercourse, especially during deep penetration, and can last for as long as 24 hours after intercourse. We are not sure why this happens, but one theory is that penetration causes pressure on endometrial deposits in the pelvis. The pain of endometriosis is related to the menstrual cycle usually building during the cycle to be at its worst just before and during a period. If you have a first degree relative (mother, sister or daughter) with the condition you are much more likely – possibly as much as nine times more likely – to have endometriosis.

It saddens me to hear that endometriosis patients wait for eight years, on average, before finally being given a diagnosis. By spending some time really thinking about your pain, hopefully, you would be diagnosed much sooner. I remember being taught that middle class, white women were more likely to suffer with endometriosis. This isn't so, but, sadly, tends to be a reflection of the fact that those women are more likely to persist in their search for an explanation and get the referral to a gynaecologist that they need. Endometriosis cannot be diagnosed with a scan or a blood test. The diagnosis is made following a procedure called a laparoscopy (a look inside with a telescope), which needs to be done under anaesthetic by a gynaecologist. There is more about endometriosis in Chapter 9.

Irritable bowel syndrome

It may seem odd that I am suddenly talking bowels when we are discussing pelvic pain, but in fact irritable bowel syndrome (IBS) is a very common cause of such pain. Food gets from your mouth, through your gut, to your rectum by being pushed along by muscular contractions in the gut wall. There is a lot of debate as to whether IBS patients have stronger than normal contractions causing the classic symptoms of cramping abdominal pain, trapped wind and bloating, and constipation or diarrhoea, or whether they simply have a heightened sensitivity to normal contractions. I suspect that both factors play a role. The pain of IBS will differ from other causes of pelvic pain, the most significant factor being the association with bowel movements. So IBS pain may cause associated diarrhoea or constipation and it is often relieved partially or completely after having your bowels open. There may be mucus in the stool and a feeling of not having completely emptied your bowels after going to the toilet. This is called **tenesmus**. There may be a link to the menstrual cycle, which is why it can be confused with a gynaecological problem. The hormonal changes just before a period can affect the muscular contractions in the bowel wall. And stress definitely plays a role – the symptoms invariably increase in times of stress and I have many patients who have medication at hand to take when the pressure is on but who manage with simple lifestyle measures, such as increasing fluid and fibre intake, when life is less stressful.

Chronic pelvic inflammatory disease

Pelvic inflammatory disease (PID) is an infection of the womb and fallopian tubes. The most common cause is a sexually transmitted infection, such as chlamydia or gonorrhoea, but it can also be caused by overgrowth of the normal bacteria living in the vagina. This is more likely after having a baby or after a procedure such as fitting a coil or having a gynaecological operation. The pain of chronic PID can be experienced on one or both sides of the pelvis and is often linked to intercourse because of sensitivity around the cervix. Some patients will give a clear story of having had a sexually transmitted infection but, as infections like chlamydia and gonorrhoea are often asymptomatic in the acute phase, it is perfectly possible to have a chronic inflammation without ever having been aware of the initial infection. There may also be an associated vaginal discharge or abnormal vaginal bleeding, which can be anything from heavier than normal periods, to bleeding after sex, or bleeding between periods.

PID can be difficult to diagnose as swabs don't always show any bacteria and scans looking for inflamed fallopian tubes may also appear normal, so it is not uncommon to need a laparoscopy to confirm the diagnosis. Treatment is usually with a combination of antibiotics but around one in five women will have a second episode of PID. This is generally because the partner wasn't treated or the course of antibiotics was not completed, so it is important that you follow the instructions of your treatment and that you practise safe sex with any new partners to reduce your risk of further problems.

Trapped ovary syndrome

This is a rare condition that occurs in about 1 in a 100 women who have had hysterectomies (removal of the womb) but where the ovaries were left in place. It occurs because the ovary gets stuck to the wall of the vagina causing pain in the pelvis, particularly during intercourse. A similar syndrome can occur in women who have had the ovaries removed at the time of hysterectomy. This is called **ovarian remnant syndrome** and is thought to be due to the presence of some functioning ovarian tissue, despite having had the ovaries removed. Both conditions can be difficult to treat, but involve surgically removing the remaining tissue.

8

Cervical disease and screening

Cervical screening

It's a common misconception that the cervical smear test is for cervical cancer. In fact the smear test is looking for changes in the cells in the cervix (the neck of the womb) that, if left, could become cancerous over a period of years. And that's why it is so important to attend for your smears when called – the smear test is designed to help prevent cancer not to diagnose it.

What does a smear test involve?

If you are registered with an NHS GP and are eligible for a smear test (see the next section) you will routinely be called, probably, to see the nurse in your practice or maybe a doctor. You will be asked to lie on your back on an examination couch, bring your knees up, keeping your ankles together, and allow your knees to fall apart. Not the most glamorous of positions but rest assured, it is all in a day's work for the person doing the test and the more relaxed you can be about it, the easier it will be for the nurse or GP to take the smear and, more importantly, the more comfortable it will be for you. A small instrument called a **speculum**, which looks a bit like the beak of a duck, will be placed into the vagina and it is then opened so that the cervix can be seen. A small plastic brush is used to sweep around the cervix, which you shouldn't be able to feel at all, and the cells that are then collected are put into a pot containing a special fluid before being sent to the laboratory for analysis under the microscope. When you have your smear, check with the smear taker, how long it will be before you get your results – it is usually a few weeks.

Who can have a smear test?

If you are registered with an NHS GP you will automatically be called for your first smear after your twenty-fifth birthday if you live in England or Northern Ireland. If you are in Wales or Scotland, it will be after your twentieth birthday. As long as everything is normal you will be called every three years until your forty-ninth birthday. After that your smears will be less frequent as the risks of abnormalities developing are reduced. So after 50 you will be called every five years until you are 65. After that you will not be called routinely, unless previous smears have been abnormal.

Why don't England and Northern Ireland call women under 25 for smear tests?

We used to screen women in England and Northern Ireland from the age of 20 and the decision to increase the age for the first smear to 25 was based on the evidence that although cervical cancer is extremely rare in women under the age of 25, abnormal results are relatively common. The vast majority of the abnormalities found in such young women revert to normal without the need for any treatment, but, of course, cause a lot of anxiety along the way. That said, it is important that sexually active women under the age of 25 know to report symptoms such as abnormal bleeding between periods or after sex, or any abnormal vaginal discharge. The vast majority of these symptoms won't be cancer at all, but symptoms like this should be checked out.

Do I have to have a smear even if I haven't ever had sex?

By far and away the most significant risk factor for developing cervical cancer is infection with the human papilloma virus, which is spread by sexual contact, but there are other, less common, types of cervical cancer so it is important you go for your smear when you are called.

Do I need to have smear if I am gay?

Just as you should still have smear tests even if you have never had sex, it is a good idea to go for your smear when you are called even if you are gay. If you have ever had heterosexual relationships, your risks are the same as anyone else, so in a nutshell – yes!

Do I need a smear if I have had a hysterectomy?

Most hysterectomies involve removing the whole of the womb including the cervix but do check with your doctor as occasionally the cervix is left. This is called a **subtotal hysterectomy** and if you have had this type of hysterectomy you will need to continue having regular smears. You will also need regular smears if you had a hysterectomy for cancer; you will need to have what we call **vault smears**, which is the same as a cervical smear but we simply take cells from the top of the vagina to check that no cancerous cells have been left in place.

Can I have a smear when I am having a period?

The best time to have a smear is mid cycle so if your appointment comes through for a time when you think you will be bleeding it is best to reschedule it. The main reason for this is that the blood may mean that not enough cells can be seen and you would just need to have the test repeated.

What do the results of a smear test mean?

Smear tests will be reported in one of three ways – normal, inadequate or abnormal.

- *Normal* Nine out of ten smears are reported as normal and this means that you will simply be called again in three or five years depending on your age. Of course, no test is 100 per cent accurate so if you should develop symptoms in between, make sure that you report them to your doctor so they can be checked out.
- *Inadequate* This simply means not enough cells were collected and you will be asked to have a repeat test. If you have three consecutive inadequate tests, you will be referred for a **colposcopy** (see the next section).
- *Abnormal* Only about 1 in 20 smears are reported as abnormal and there are varying degrees of abnormality from a borderline case to invasive disease. It is important to remember that the vast majority of abnormal smears are *not* cancerous and nine out of ten significant changes, known as **dyskaryosis**, actually revert back to normal without the need for treatment. Most abnormal smear results will simply mean that you are asked to attend for a repeat smear at a shorter time interval to check that the changes are resolving. If the abnormalities are more severe, or if changes don't improve on their own, you will be referred for a colposcopy.

What is a colposcopy?

A colposcopy is a more detailed look at the cervix. It is usually done in outpatients by a trained doctor or nurse. You will be asked to lie on an examination couch and your feet will be put into stirrups. A speculum is used, just like for a normal smear test, but instead of looking at the cervix directly the doctor or nurse uses a special telescope called a **colposcope**. This doesn't go inside you but is placed between your legs. A special liquid is used to paint the cervix, which helps to highlight any abnormal cells, but you won't feel that and a small sample of tissue is taken from the cervix for more in-depth analysis in the laboratory. The whole thing should only take about 15 minutes and you will be given a follow-up appointment to decide whether any further treatment is required once the results are available.

What is the human papilloma virus?

There are over 100 different types of human papilloma virus (HPV). Some cause warts and verrucas, others are responsible for changes in the cervix that can lead to cervical cancer. In fact the association between HPV infection and cervical cancer is so strong that it is thought that 99 per cent of cases of cervical cancer are caused by infection with the high-risk HPV types 16 and 18. The virus is spread by sexual contact and is so common that around half of British adults will be infected at some point in their lives. For most of us this causes no problems at all. There are no symptoms associated with the infection and our immune system simply clears the virus within a couple of years but in some cases the infection persists, causing pre-cancerous cells in the cervix. There is now a vaccine against the high-risk strains of HPV that is offered to all girls in Britain aged 12 and 13. It is given as three separate injections over a period of six months. The thinking behind offering it so young is to vaccinate the girls before they become sexually active and, therefore, prevent infection with the virus.

Cervical cancer

Cervical cancer is a largely preventable disease. In 99 per cent of cases, infection with HPV is to blame. Now that we have an effective vaccination against this virus, and as long as women attend for their smears when called, we should be able to all but eradicate the disease. Today, around a thousand women die each year of cervical cancer. This disease is most common in women in their 30s and 40s, so anything we can do to reduce that number has to be a priority. Women who smoke and anyone with a suppressed immune system, such as those with AIDS or people taking immune suppressant medication, are more at risk, and there has been a slight increase in risk seen in women who have taken the combined oral contraceptive pill for more than eight years.

What are the symptoms of cervical cancer?

There may be no symptoms at all in the early stages, which is why it is so important that women attend for their smears so that pre-cancerous changes can be picked up and dealt with. If symptoms do develop, they may include abnormal discharge or bleeding such as bleeding after sex, between periods, or after the menopause. These symptoms are relatively common and in the majority of cases due to much less serious problems, but they should never be ignored.

What happens if I am diagnosed with cervical cancer?

If you are diagnosed with cervical cancer, the first thing your doctors will want to do is to find out how far the cancer has spread as this will determine what is the best treatment for you. This may involve blood tests, X-rays, ultrasounds and MRI scans. If caught early, treatment will aim to cure the cancer and will almost certainly involve surgery to remove the womb and cervix. This means that the option of bearing children naturally in the future is now an impossibility, which is, of course, devastating to women who have not finished (or, in some instances, not even started) their families but the surgery can be life saving. You may also be offered radiotherapy and chemotherapy.

Cervical polyps and erosions

Cervical polyps are benign lumps that arise in the cervical canal. They are often just noted on a routine examination, for example during a cervical smear, but if they do cause any symptoms, the symptom is most likely to be abnormal bleeding. The polyps look like small red cherries at the opening of the cervix and, as they are usually attached via a stalk, they can often be removed by simply twisting them around. I have removed lots of these in my consulting room without the patient feeling anything, but occasionally they are more tricky and need to be removed in hospital, under local or general anaesthetic. They are very rarely cancerous so are usually nothing to worry about.

Cervical erosions are extremely common and look like red patches on the cervix. They are so common that if I see one in women of childbearing age, or in a lady who is on the combined contraceptive pill, it wouldn't even warrant comment. But if they do cause problems it is likely to be abnormal bleeding, particularly after intercourse, or a vaginal discharge. If this is the case they can usually be managed by painting the cervix with a special paint. You may need a second treatment a couple of weeks later and you may be advised to consider an alternative form of contraception if you are on the combined pill.

9

Endometrial disease

Endometrial cancer

You may never even have thought about cancer of the womb; it isn't common so, unlike breast cancer, you may not know anyone who has suffered with the condition. It affects around eight thousand women in the UK each year and is mostly seen in women over 50. The more exposure to oestrogen that a woman has had during her lifetime, the greater the risk of developing the condition. So the earlier you start your periods and the later you go through the menopause the greater the risk. Being overweight will also increase your chances of developing endometrial cancer, as fat cells generate oestrogen; and women who never have children are also at risk. There is a small increased risk for diabetics, those taking tamoxifen (a breast cancer drug) and women with polycystic ovary syndrome. Interestingly there are fewer cases of endometrial cancer in Eastern countries and some people think that a western diet, which is high in fat, may also pose a risk.

What do I need to look out for?

The most common symptom of endometrial cancer is bleeding after going through the menopause, so no post-menopausal bleed should be ignored. I have lost count of the number of endometrial biopsy tests I have done to investigate post-menopausal bleeding and, thankfully, I can count the cases of endometrial cancer these tests have picked up on the fingers of one hand, so don't panic if you start bleeding after going through the change but don't ignore it either.

Other symptoms include bleeding after sex or between periods, pain during or after sex, and an unexplained vaginal discharge.

How is endometrial cancer diagnosed?

If your doctor wants to rule out the possibility of endometrial cancer they will arrange for you to have an endometrial biopsy test. This involves passing a small straw-like device through the neck of the womb to collect some cells using gentle suction. These cells are then analysed under a microscope to look for abnormalities. You may also have an ultrasound test to look at the thickness of the lining of the womb – this may be done with a probe on the lower abdomen or via the vagina, but either way it should be completely painless. It may also be suggested that you have a hysteroscopy where a small telescope is inserted into the womb to look at the lining directly, and if any areas look abnormal samples of tissue can be removed for further analysis.

Like all cancers it is important to establish the spread of the disease before deciding on a treatment plan so if you are faced with a diagnosis you will then be given further tests including blood tests, X-rays and scans to look at how far the cancer has spread.

Can endometrial cancer be cured?

Like all cancers the earlier it is detected, the better the outlook and if caught before it has spread outside the womb then surgery to remove the womb is usually curative. The good thing about endometrial cancer, if there can be a good thing about cancer, is that the symptoms of abnormal bleeding usually present quite early on in the disease, so as long as they are not ignored, the outlook for endometrial cancer is generally quite good. If the disease has already spread at the time of diagnosis a cure is less likely, but still possible, and you may be offered radiotherapy and chemotherapy.

Endometriosis

Endometrium is the medical term for the lining of the womb and endometriosis describes a condition where this tissue is found outside the womb, most commonly elsewhere in the pelvis, but it can be anywhere in the body. No one really knows why this happens – one theory is that when the womb lining is shed during a period that some endometrial cells flow backwards along the fallopian tube to settle in the pelvis. The cells in this tissue are still responsive to the hormones that drive our menstrual cycle so they will proliferate each month on the build up to a period and can cause the classic symptoms of pelvic pain, and often pain during intercourse, as they feel tender during penetration.

There are various figures bandied about as to how common the condition is but, as so many women suffer in silence, I think it is impossible to know for sure. I have met several women who have only been diagnosed following investigation for subfertility or when the deposits of endometrial tissue are found during surgery, such as a caesarean section. The condition typically develops between the ages of 25 and 40 and there is sometimes a family history.

What are the symptoms of endometriosis?

Some women will have no symptoms whatsoever – these are the ones we only diagnose as a chance finding during investigation or surgery for something else – but if symptoms do occur, the most common are painful periods; the pain is often more severe than normal period pain and tends to last throughout the period rather than wearing off after the first few days. Pain during sex is also common and can last for several hours after intercourse. Because the deposits of endometriosis are often sticky like congealing blood they can cause what we call adhesions where organs stick together; for example, part of the bowel may stick to the outside of the womb or the wall of the pelvis causing more persistent pain. Endometriosis can sometimes cause problems with fertility.

How is endometriosis diagnosed?

Endometriosis can't be diagnosed with a blood test or a scan. To confirm the presence of endometrial deposits in the pelvis, you will need to have a procedure called a laparoscopy. This is where a small telescope is inserted into your tummy via a cut around your tummy button to look directly into the pelvis. This has to be done under general anaesthetic because the gynaecologist will need to inflate your tummy with gas to separate the bowel and give a good view. This can cause irritation of the diaphragm, which can cause pain in the shoulder. So don't be surprised if you notice shoulder pain the day after this procedure – it settles very quickly.

How is endometriosis treated?

Not everyone will need treatment. If symptoms are mild, simple painkillers may be all that is required and in about a third of cases the symptoms will resolve without any treatment at all. Unfortunately, for some women the symptoms get worse over time, and then we need to treat more aggressively. The first line of treatment is probably to try taking the combined oral contraceptive pill. We know that the pill works by preventing ovulation and women on the pill tend to have lighter and shorter periods, which is probably why it helps in some women with endometriosis. There is also something called the **intra-uterine system**, which is like a coil in the womb, but it secretes tiny amounts of hormone into the womb lining (about the same as taking two mini pills a week). Most women stop their periods altogether when this is fitted so it helps with the pain of endometriosis. Progestogens can also be taken orally to counteract the effects of oestrogen. There are other medicines which act on the pituitary gland in the brain to stop it from producing the hormones that drive the ovaries. All of these treatments can reduce fertility, which is an issue for some women who want to start or increase their families, and for these women, and in severe cases, surgery is an option. The deposits can be removed surgically or by laser.

Fibroids

Fibroids are non-cancerous tumours made up of muscle and fibrous tissue that grow in or around the womb. They are extremely common – around half of all 50 year olds will have fibroids and most won't cause any problems. If they do cause symptoms, the most common will be heavy periods but, depending on the size of the fibroid, they can also cause symptoms related to the pressure they put on surrounding tissues. Larger fibroids can cause pain during intercourse, constipation, or the need to wee more frequently. We don't really know why they form but we do know that they are oestrogen dependent so they are more common in overweight women, because they have higher levels of oestrogen, and will shrink after the menopause when oestrogen levels fall.

How are fibroids treated?

If fibroids are not causing symptoms then no treatment is necessary. If heavy periods are a problem you may be offered an intra-uterine system, which is like a coil that secretes tiny doses of progestogen into the womb to reduce bleeding. Alternatively, non-hormonal prescription medicines called tranexamic or mefenamic acid can reduce bleeding by up to 50 per cent. The combined pill may also help as it tends to cause lighter periods. There are also injections called **gonadotropin releasing hormone analogues** that reduce oestrogen levels and, therefore, help shrink fibroids. They can only be used for six months at a time and unfortunately the fibroids may regrow when treatment stops. Large fibroids may need surgery. If you have finished your family, you may opt for a hysterectomy but there are alternatives.

- *Endometrial ablation* This is usually a day-case procedure where the lining of the womb is removed using laser, microwave technology, a heated loop or hot fluid in a balloon. The procedure takes about 20 minutes and you may feel some discomfort for a few days and notice a vaginal discharge, but most women are back to work within a fortnight.
- *Myomectomy* This is done either by keyhole surgery or through a larger cut in your tummy to remove fibroids from the wall of the womb. Not all fibroids can be removed this way and your gynaecologist will tell you if this is a suitable option for you.
- *Uterine artery embolization* This involves injecting a chemical under X-ray control into the blood vessels that supply the fibroid. It is done under local anaesthetic and usually involves staying in hospital for a day or two.
- *Hysteroscopic resection* This involves using a telescope inserted via the vagina, through the cervical canal, into the womb. Instruments are then passed through the hysteroscope and used to remove the fibroids. This is also usually a day-case procedure and is suitable for small fibroids.
- *MRI-guided techniques* This is cutting edge technology. MRI is used to guide small needles into the middle of the fibroid and then laser or ultrasound energy is passed through the needles to destroy the fibroid.

10

Ovarian disease

Ovarian cancer

It often surprises women when they hear that ovarian cancer is more common than cervical cancer. It is in fact the fifth most common cancer in women in the UK. There are three different types of ovarian cancer, but by far the most common form, accounting for 90 per cent of all ovarian cancers, is what we call **epithelial ovarian cancer** where the cancer forms in the cells surrounding the ovary. Other forms arise from the cells that make the eggs (**germ cell ovarian cancer**) or the cells that produce the hormones (**stromal ovarian cancer**).

What causes epithelial ovarian cancer?

There is no one specific cause but most cases occur after the menopause, so increasing age is a definite risk factor. Anything that increases oestrogen exposure will also increase the risk – so being overweight or obese, not having children, having a late menopause or taking HRT are all risk factors for ovarian cancer. In a minority of cases (about one in ten) there is a genetic component – carriers of the *BRCA1* and *BRCA2* genes are at increased risk. If you have a strong family history of breast and ovarian cancer at a young age, it is worth talking to your GP about being tested for these genes. You will need to have counselling because, of course, there will be some major decisions to be made if you test positive.

What are the symptoms of ovarian cancer?

Sadly, ovarian cancer has been called the silent killer because the early symptoms may be vague and attributed to other, much more common, conditions – typically IBS. If you have a family history of ovarian cancer, it is important that you take note of the early symptoms and report them to your GP. Constant pain in the pelvis and persistent bloating should not be ignored, and it is the persistence that is key. We all get bloated from time to time, but if it doesn't settle, and particularly if it is associated with a feeling of being full very quickly, it should be checked out. Ovarian cancer may also make your tummy look distended. It can cause you to lose weight. The pressure effects may mean that you need to pass water more frequently, or cause you to be constipated. You may also experience pain in the lower abdomen or in your back.

Why don't we screen for ovarian cancer like we do for breast and cervical cancer?

For a screening test to be useful it must be sensitive enough to pick up as many cases as possible and mustn't flag up too many of what we call **false positives**. The smear test looking for pre-cancerous cells on the cervix, and the mammogram for breast cancer, fulfil these criteria well. Work is being done on a screening test which could include an ultrasound and a blood test looking for a protein called *CA-125,*which is raised in ovarian cancer. The outlook for ovarian cancer would be massively improved if we could find a way of detecting the disease earlier, but at the moment the tests aren't specific enough to use in all women as too many tests would give false positive results and some women would end up undergoing unnecessary surgery. That said, women who have two or more close relatives who have had pre-menopausal breast cancer or ovarian cancer may be offered the tests that we currently have available, as their risk is significantly higher than that of the general population.

How is ovarian cancer treated?

Before treatment is decided, the disease must be staged (see Chapter 1), which involves scans to check whether the disease is confined to the ovary (Stage 1), whether it has spread to other areas of the pelvis (Stage 2), whether it has spread beyond the pelvis (Stage 3) or whether it has spread to other organs, such as the liver and lungs (Stage 4). Stage 1 disease can be treated surgically by removing the ovary and fallopian tube; Stage 2 disease may also require surgery but more tissue will be removed and the gynaecologist will probably also take samples of tissue from elsewhere in the pelvis and from lymph nodes to check whether the disease has spread further than is initially obvious. Chemotherapy is sometimes given before surgery to try to shrink the tumour before the operation, and while radiotherapy is not generally used to treat ovarian cancer, it is sometimes given after surgery to try to kill any cancer cells that may have been left after the operation.

Polycystic ovary syndrome

The diagnosis of polycystic ovary syndrome (PCOS) is made in women who have at least two of the following three problems:

1 Raised testosterone levels – all women have small amounts of the male hormone testosterone but in polycystic ovary syndrome (PCOS) these levels are raised;
2 Multiple (at least 12) cysts in the ovaries;
3 Anovulatory cycles i.e. menstrual cycles where ovulation does not occur.

The underlying problems explain the wide variety of symptoms associated with the syndrome: the raised testosterone levels may cause acne, unwanted facial or body hair and thinning of the scalp hair; the anovulatory cycles may lead to erratic periods and problems with fertility.

PCOS sufferers become resistant to insulin meaning that insulin levels rise and high insulin levels lead to weight gain. This becomes something of a vicious circle as excess fat makes insulin resistance worse and the circulating insulin levels rise further still, meaning further potential weight gain. In the long term, PCOS increases the risk of developing type 2 diabetes, high blood pressure and high cholesterol. Unsurprisingly, lots of women with PCOS develop issues with low self-esteem and some become depressed.

How is PCOS treated?

It is tough for women with PCOS to lose weight because of the high circulating insulin levels, but weight loss is vital as it will improve so many of the associated symptoms. Losing weight will help reduce insulin levels and testosterone levels, which means the problems with acne and unwanted hair start to improve. It also means you are more likely to ovulate. You may be prescribed a diabetic drug called metformin which makes the body more sensitive to insulin so ultimately reduces insulin levels, which helps with weight loss. As I have said weight loss will help improve the other . symptoms, but if facial hair continues to be a problem this can be removed by waxing, shaving or plucking. If you have dark hair, bleaching the unwanted hair may also improve its appearance. For a more long term solution, electrolysis or laser are very effective. Laser isn't cheap, but it is particularly effective on dark hair and can produce an excellent result.

There is a contraceptive pill called Dianette that is effective at treating facial hair and acne and there is also a cream available on prescription called eflornithine, which work on an enzyme in the hair follicle to prevent regrowth of the hair. In some areas, eflornithine is categorised as 'Not normally funded', so your GP would have to make a special case to prescribe it for you on the NHS. The idea is that you remove any unwanted hair in your normal way and then if this cream is used every day the hair does not grow back. You do have to persevere though because, as soon as you stop using the cream, the hair will regrow.

Acne can be treated in the usual way with antibiotic creams or tablets, and prescription medicines called retinoids. Losing weight helps with fertility issues but some women require a procedure to drill into the ovaries to help with fertility.

11

Vulval disease

Vulval cancer

Cancer can occur anywhere in the body. When it occurs on the vulva it tends to occur on the inner surface of the vulval lips known as the **labia minora** and **labia majora**, but it can also occur on the skin around the lips of the vulva or in the clitoris. Vulval cancer is rare – there are around 1,000 new cases each year in the UK and it almost always develops after the menopause. There is no one specific cause but we do know that there are some things that increase your risk of developing the disease.

What are the risk factors for developing vulval cancer?

Age Vulval cancer is extremely rare in pre-menopausal women. Most cases occur after the age of 55.

Human papilloma virus I have already discussed the role of HPV in the development of cervical cancer and it would seem that it plays a similar role in the development of vulval cancer. HPV types 16, 18 and 31 increase the risk of developing a condition called **vulval intra-epithelial neoplasia** (VIN) and around a third of all vulval cancers develop from VIN. HPV only seems to play a part in developing vulval cancer in approximately 50 per cent of all cases, whereas it is responsible for 99 per cent of cervical cancers.

Smoking Smoking depresses the immune system making it less likely that you will effectively clear HPV from your system.

Lichen sclerosus and lichen planus Both these conditions cause inflammation and irritation of the skin around the vulva and in a small number of women this can lead to vulval cancer.

Genital herpes Herpes infection is very common and in most cases has no link to cancer; in a small minority of women it can increase the risk of developing vulval cancer.

What should I look out for?

The most common symptom of vulval cancer is a persistent itch or soreness. Some women describe a burning sensation, especially when passing urine. It may not be a part of your body that you are used to examining but using a mirror, either sitting on the floor or with one foot on a chair, you can look at the skin around the vulva. Thickened or raised areas, persistent ulcers or areas of discolouration – either darker looking skin or patches of lighter looking skin – should always be checked out. Any unusual swelling, or having a mole in that area that is changing, should also be reported. Most vulval cancers develop in the skin cells themselves, but about 4 per cent develop in the pigment cells and may present as a changing mole. The changes you are looking for are any difference in the size, shape or colour, or a mole that starts to itch or bleed.

How is vulval cancer treated?

The diagnosis will first be confirmed by taking a small biopsy of tissue under local anaesthetic for examination under a microscope. If you have vulval cancer your specialist will probably then want to arrange various blood tests and scans to assess how far the cancer has spread before deciding on the best treatment for you. You will almost certainly be offered surgery in the first instance, unless the cancer is widely spread and your general health is such that surgery may not be the best option for you. Exactly what operation you will have will depend on the size and position of the cancer. Smaller cancers may be treated by removing just the abnormal area and a small amount of surrounding tissue, whereas larger cancers may involve removing the entire vulval area – the labia minora, majora and clitoris. Radiotherapy my be another option – as most vulval cancers develop in skin cells and are squamous cell cancers they are usually sensitive to radiotherapy. Chemotherapy may also be an option.

Lichen sclerosus

Lichen sclerosus affects about 1 in a 1000 women and causes itching around the genital area. We don't know what causes lichen sclerosus and, sadly, we don't have a cure as yet. It can last for years, causing a lot of angst and discomfort. It usually starts as small white spots around the vulva that are intensely itchy. Over time these spots may join together to form larger patches of white skin. Because they are so itchy, the trauma from scratching means that the skin may split and bleed and, if left untreated, the resulting scar tissue may mean that the entrance to the vagina becomes narrower, making inter-course more difficult. Regular use of steroid ointment, on prescription from your doctor, will alleviate the symptoms but it should be used sparingly – as a rough guide a 30 g tube of steroid ointment should last around three months.

What else can I do to help myself?

If you have lichen sclerosis, try not to scratch the area. So much easier to say than to do, but the more you scratch, the more you traumatise the skin and the worse the itching becomes so you end up in a vicious scratch–itch cycle. Keep your nails short and wear cotton gloves in bed so that you don't damage the skin in your sleep by scratching before you are fully awake. An antihistamine at night may also help. Avoid anything perfumed in that area – so no bubble baths or perfumed soap as these may irritate the skin further. Use aqueous cream as a soap substitute. It won't lather in the same way but is very effective and helps soothe the skin. Use an emollient such as petroleum jelly on the area before passing urine to protect from the stinging, only wear natural fibres, and wear stockings rather than tights to keep you cool, as sweating increases the itching. If you are aware that sex is becoming uncomfortable, you will need to use plenty of lubricant and speak to your doctor about vaginal dilators to keep the area open.

Lichen planus

Lichen planus also causes itching, but it can affect other areas of the body, including the limbs, mouth, nails and scalp, as well as the genitals. Unlike lichen sclerosis it tends to clear up after several months and rarely lasts more than 18 months. Steroid creams will help with symptoms, as will all the self-help measures used to manage lichen sclerosis.

Bartholin's cysts

The Bartholin's glands are small, pea-sized glands that sit just inside the vagina; their function is to secrete lubricant fluid during intercourse. Sometimes the ducts that deliver the fluid can become blocked and the cyst develops. Small cysts may not cause any problems at all and, although any new lump should be checked out by your doctor, you may not need any specific treatment. Sometimes if the cysts become very large, they can be painful and interfere with sex, in which case they may need to be removed surgically although, in about one in five cases, they do recur. If they become sore and inflamed this could suggest infection which will need antibiotics.

12

Vaginal discharge and sexually transmitted infections

Reasons for changes in vaginal discharge

All women will experience vaginal discharge. The vaginal discharge will be different for every woman, and vaginal discharge also varies throughout the cycle for each woman. It is thought that around one in ten women will consult their GP during their lifetime with concerns over vaginal discharge, and what is normal for one woman may not be acceptable for another. Sometimes the woman will simply be looking for reassurance that everything is healthy, but sometimes abnormal vaginal discharge may be related to a problem, such as thrush, bacterial vaginosis (BV) or some sexually transmitted infections (STIs), that needs further investigation or treatment.

What is normal vaginal discharge?

Normal vaginal discharge is colourless or white, although it may become more yellow on exposure to air as a result of oxidation. It should not be blood stained and should not have an odour. It tends to become thicker and more profuse following ovulation, and some women using oral contraception or the coil may notice an increase in the amount of discharge they produce. A change in your vaginal secretions doesn't necessarily mean infection. A cervical erosion or polyp can cause increased discharge and a foreign body in the vagina – most commonly a forgotten tampon – is a relatively common cause of discharge. Occasionally, it can also be a sign of a cancer but this is extremely rare and infective causes are much more likely.

Thrush

Thrush is caused by a yeast called *Candida albicans*, which is actually present in the vagina of 20 per cent of all women without causing symptoms. If it does cause symptoms, it is likely to cause soreness and itching in the vagina and vulva and a cottage cheese-like discharge.

Who gets thrush?

Thrush is extremely common and there may be no obvious reason why some women get it frequently, but it is more common in some groups.

- *Diabetes* Diabetics with poor diabetic control will have high blood sugar levels that provide the perfect environment for thrush to thrive. In fact, if a woman presents with recurrent thrush she should always be tested for undiagnosed diabetes.
- *Pregnancy* Hormonal changes in pregnancy can increase the likelihood of developing thrush.
- *Antibiotics* It is normal to have bacteria in our vaginas and, when in the right balance, these bacteria play a role in keeping the vagina clean and healthy. If you have antibiotics for an infection elsewhere in the body, that can reduce the amount of bacteria in your vagina meaning that the yeast that causes thrush can proliferate to cause symptoms.
- *Steroids* Taking steroids increases the likelihood of developing thrush.
- *Immune problems* AIDS or taking drugs to damp down your immune system, for other conditions you may have, can make you more prone to thrush.

Contrary to popular belief, taking the combined oral contraceptive pill has not been proven to make you more prone to thrush, but if I see a woman plagued with recurrent thrush who is using the combined pill, I sometimes suggest an alternative form of contraception and occasionally this does the trick.

Will I have to have a swab test?

I don't always swab women with symptoms of thrush. If you have had it before, recognize the symptoms, and are in a monogamous relationship you may simply need the treatment, which can come in the form of creams, pessaries or tablets. If, however, there is any possibility of a sexually transmitted infection your doctor will want to check this out with a swab test.

What can I do to prevent thrush developing?

If you suffer with recurrent thrush, make sure you only use underwear made with natural fibres. Avoid man-made fibres, which are likely to make you sweat, and, wherever possible, keep clothing loose. Try to avoid any perfumed products as this will alter the naturally acidic environment of the vagina and mean that the yeast can thrive. The yeast that causes thrush grows in the bowel so after going to the toilet always wipe front to back to avoid encouraging the yeast forward to the vaginal opening. Thrush is not a sexually transmitted infection but some women notice flares after sexual intercourse – if this is you, make sure you use plenty of lubricant during sex to reduce any trauma to the delicate vaginal skin. I often recommend a daily probiotic to maintain good gut health and keep the yeast in balance too. If you suffer with recurrent thrush your doctor may suggest a longer course of treatment in the form of an antifungal tablet taken once a week for four weeks.

Bacterial vaginosis

Just as thrush is caused by an overgrowth of yeast, BV is caused by an overgrowth of a bacteria called *Gardnerella vaginalis* that occurs naturally in the vagina. It is actually twice as common as thrush although in my experience many women have never heard of it and it is important to know of its existence. I have met so many women over the years who have been self-treating what they presume to be thrush when in fact they have BV.

How can I tell the difference between thrush and BV?

The only way to be absolutely sure is to have a swab test, but there are some characteristic differences. The discharge of thrush tends to be thick and white, like cottage cheese, while the discharge of BV is likely to be more watery and grey; however, the main difference is the odour. The discharge of BV has a fishy odour which women find extremely embarrassing and distressing. Itching is much more a symptom of thrush than BV.

How is bacterial vaginosis treated?

Unlike thrush, BV is treated with antibiotics either by mouth or as a vaginal cream. This can, of course, mean you are more prone to thrush and I have met some poor women who seem to oscillate between the two infections. In these women, I recommend using a lactic acid gel inserted into the vagina to maintain a healthy vaginal pH and keep the bacteria in balance. It is particularly important to treat BV in pregnant women as it has been linked to miscarriage and premature birth.

Sexually transmitted infections

Chlamydia

I am discussing chlamydia in the context of vaginal discharge and sexually transmitted infection, but perhaps the first thing to say is that at least 70 per cent of women with chlamydia will have no symptoms at all and those that do have symptoms may only have a mild discharge. Other symptoms include bleeding between periods, pelvic or lower abdominal pain, or pain on passing urine. In fact if a woman presents to me with bleeding between periods, which cannot be explained by missed pills, or any other obvious cause, it is chlamydia until proved otherwise.

Unfortunately, chlamydia is so prevalent because it often goes unrecognized and I have met too many women over the years who only discover they have been infected when they are trying for a baby and discover that previously undiagnosed chlamydia has resulted in blocked fallopian tubes, leading to infertility. Like all things, prevention is better than cure – practising safe sex by using a barrier method of contraception with new sexual partners will protect you from this disease.

Gonorrhoea

While gonorrhoea can go undetected, like chlamydia, it is more likely to cause symptoms. Around 50 per cent of women with gonorrhoea will notice a change in their vaginal discharges and, just like chlamydia, if left untreated it can have implications for future fertility. So if you know you have been at possible risk, it is worth getting checked out. Treatment of both conditions requires a simple course of antibiotics.

Trichomoniasis

The discharge of trichomoniasis is frothy. It may smell fishy, just like BV but, unlike BV, soreness and irritation can be quite intense. Just like chlamydia and gonorrhoea, it may show no symptoms at all. It is easily treated with antibiotics and it is important that it is treated because the presence of trichomoniasis can increase your risk of contracting HIV and, if caught during pregnancy, it increases the risk of premature labour.

Genital warts

Genital warts remain the most common STI. They are caused by infection with HPV types 6 and 11. These are not the strains of HPV that are implicated in cervical and other forms of cancer, but they are covered by the vaccine that is currently offered to all 12 and 13 year old girls so we will hopefully see a fall in the incidence of genital warts in the future. Genital warts are spread by skin to skin contact, so the use of condoms doesn't offer full protection. The warts can develop a few weeks after contact, but can also be noticed for the first time several years after infection so the recent onset of warts doesn't necessarily mean a partner has been unfaithful!

Small warts may be treated by the application of creams or ointments for a few days each week, sometimes for several weeks. They can be frozen off by cryotherapy, or removed by heat using electrocautery. They can also removed surgically under local anaesthetic or by using a laser.

Genital herpes

Genital herpes is the most common cause of ulcers on the genitals and these can be extremely painful. There are two types of herpes simplex virus – types 1 and 2. Usually, type 1 causes cold sores and type 2 causes genital ulceration, but there is quite a bit of overlap and either type can cause either symptom.

The first episode of herpes often involves multiple ulcers, which are painful and can last up to three weeks. These can be treated with antiviral medication on prescription. Subsequent attacks are, thankfully, typically less severe and often heralded by a tingling sensation. If antiviral cream available over the counter is used at this stage, the blisters can be avoided. Once an individual has contracted herpes, the infection never completely clears from the body. The virus crawls back up the nerve endings and lays dormant.

In some people, there will never be a recurrence but, for some, recurrences are a regular problem. They tend to flare when you are run down or stressed, and after exposure to ultra violet light. During a flare up, you will be highly infectious and should avoid sexual intercourse. Once the lesions have healed you are of very low infectivity, but it is still possible to pass the virus on so condoms should be used all the time.

Syphilis

Syphilis is a sexually transmitted infection caused by a bacteria called *Treponema pallidum*. The first stage of the disease, known as **primary syphilis**, causes painless ulcers on the genital area. These usually occur two to three weeks after the infection was caught and are highly infectious. They can take up to six weeks to heal. The second stage, known as **secondary syphilis**, causes a painless non-itchy pink or red rash all over the body. There may also be warty-like lesions around the vulva which can easily be mistaken for warts and white patches on the roof of the mouth along with patchy hair loss. The third stage, or **tertiary syphilis**, is very rare in the UK and occurs several years later, causing damage to the heart, bones brain and nervous system. Syphilis is easily treated with antibiotic injections. In primary and secondary syphilis this treatment will completely cure the condition. You can also cure tertiary syphilis quickly, but you cannot reverse the damage already done to the heart, bones, brain or nerves.

13

Sexual problems

Normal sexual function

I hesitate to use the word *normal* here because of course every woman's experience of sexual function is very personal and can vary from day to day and throughout life. What is normal and fulfilling for one woman may not be for the next, but bear with me while I try to talk through what I see as the four stages of female sexual function.

Sexual desire or libido Few women would argue that the female libido is complex. I have a friend who lectures regularly on the subject. The female libido she likens to a remote control. There are 20 or 30 buttons with labels for everything including 'Time of the month' to 'Work stress', 'Kids' homework' and 'How tidy is the house?'. She always gets a laugh, and goes on to say that not only is the remote very complex but that in order for the right channel to be selected, the buttons need to be pressed in a particular order! She gets a further laugh when she shows the male remote, which simply reads 'Beer' and 'Sex'!

Arousal The initial response to sexual stimulation is vascular dilation, allowing engorgement of the genital tissues, followed by changes in the nerves and muscles that allow the vagina to balloon and the clitoris to retract slightly.

Orgasm The muscles around the vagina contract and the woman feels a sensation of climax.

Resolution During this phase all the changes described above gradually reverse.

Low libido

This is probably the most common sexual problem that I see in surgery. There are two main different types, which in medicine we refer to as **primary low sexual desire** and **secondary low sexual desire**. As the name implies, primary low sexual desire refers to the woman who has never had an interest in sexual activity. There are usually deep-rooted issues behind this – often a woman with primary low sexual desire will have been brought up being told that sex is wrong or dirty, and unravelling that can take a lot of time in therapy. Secondary low sexual desire is the more common problem and refers to the woman who has had a healthy sex drive in the past, but has lost all interest in recent weeks, months or years. By the time I see women like this in my consulting room, it has usually been an issue for months or years and, more often than not, she has been encouraged to seek help by her partner. The first question to ask yourself is whether you ever have any sexual desire. If you masturbate or have sexual fantasies but have no sexual interest in your partner then you are looking at a relationship issue and that needs to be addressed.

It is common for women to notice a drop in their libido following childbirth and this is down to several factors. Your hormones are all over the place. Your body will have changed shape, and you may feel less attractive. I always encourage women who are bothered by this to invest in some new underwear that fits and makes them feel better about themselves. It takes time to regain a pre-pregnancy figure, and most of us never return completely to the pre-pregnancy state, but remember it is a small price to pay for the wonder that is motherhood and, in time, you will learn to be comfortable in your new body. You are also likely to be tired. Bed becomes for sleeping in when you are experiencing sleepless nights, so don't be too hard on yourself. When your baby starts to sleep through, and you actually manage to get some sleep again, your libido will return but it is not uncommon for women to notice a fall in their libido for up to a year after childbirth.

Another time in life when I see a lot of women experiencing a fall in their sexual desire is around the time of the menopause. For some women this is an emotional time and comes with the realization that they are getting older, which influences how they feel sexually. Vaginal dryness is also extremely common around this time and can make sex uncomfortable or sometimes even painful. Let's face it – sex is supposed to be fun and if it hurts then it is completely natural to go off the idea! The sadness for me is that so few women report this symptom. More often than not it is a conversation that we have when I notice the tissues of the vagina look a little thin and dry and I ask the question of whether sex is uncomfortable directly. I am usually given one of several responses – 'I can't remember the last time we had sex', 'Yes, it is actually but my husband is very understanding' or 'Yes – it's a bit of an issue actually' – yet very few women proactively come in to ask for help because they assume it is just something they have to put up with as they get older. NO!

Oestrogen pessaries or vaginal cream are very effective at treating this and don't carry the risks of conventional HRT as they are only used in the vagina. When they are first used some hormone does get absorbed into the body through the thin vaginal tissues but as they start to work, the vaginal tissues plump up and become lubricated again and this prevents the absorption of hormone into the body. So it is not uncommon to notice some hormonal symptoms such as breast tenderness and bloating in the early stages but this will subside as the pessaries or cream start to work. Some women really don't want to consider anything hormonal but there are plenty of slow-release lubricants available to help alleviate the problem and your pharmacist will be able to advise you. Pharmacies have confidential consulting rooms now so all you have to do is to ask to speak the pharmacist privately. You don't have to talk about this over the counter in front of other people.

Pain during intercourse

Pain during intercourse is a common problem and to identify the cause, your doctor will want to know:

- Is the pain at the entrance to the vagina?
- Is the pain felt deep inside?
- Is intercourse painful all the time or just in certain positions?

Pain at the entrance to the vagina can be due to a condition called **vaginismus** (see the next section) where the muscles around the entrance go into spasm as soon as penetration is attempted. It can also be due to a condition called **vulvo-dynia** where the tissues around the entrance become over sensitive; this is often triggered by an infection which may be something as simple as thrush. This can be treated with creams available on prescription from your GP.

Sometimes there is a small tear to explain the pain, or scar tissue that is not as elastic as healthy vaginal tissue. This can happen following a tear or an episiotomy during childbirth. If there is scar tissue, your doctor may suggest you see a gynaecologist to discuss the option of excising the scar and refashioning it, which often gives good results.

Pain deeper in the vagina which is only felt in certain posi- tions is likely to be due to very deep penetration and can be managed by explaining this to your partner and avoiding those positions. If it occurs during all sexual activity it is more likely to be related to a problem in the pelvis such as endometriosis or chronic PID. It surprises women to know that sometimes it can be due to IBS. The important thing is that you shouldn't put up with it. Once your doctor has worked out what is causing the pain he or she will be able to refer you to someone who can help.

Vaginismus

Vaginismus is spasm of the muscles around the entrance to the vagina, which causes pain on attempted penetration. When severe, it makes penetration impossible. Most cases are primary – that is, it has always been a problem – but it can also be secondary; for example, following trauma during intercourse or a bad sexual experience, such as rape. Treatment involves a combination of psychosexual counselling and the use of vaginal dilators. These come in a variety of sizes so that a woman can start by inserting the smallest cone into her vagina by herself in private, and, over time, gradually working up to the larger cones, which are the size of the average erect penis. It can take several months before full penetrative sex is enjoyable but, with the support of psychosexual counselling, some great results are possible.

Index